GUIDE TO UNDERSTANDING SCLERODERMA
STEPS TO MANAGING AND LIVING WITH AUTOIMMUNE DISEASE

Dr.Philip.G.Rhode

TABLE OF CONTENT

Chapter 1

Introduction to scleroderma:
Although uncommon, scleroderma is a chronic autoimmune condition in which normal tissue is replaced by dense, thick fibrous tissue. Typically, the resistant framework safeguards the body against sickness and contamination. The immune system causes other cells in patients with scleroderma to produce an excessive amount of collagen (a protein). The skin and organs harden and thicken as a result of this extra collagen being deposited there, similar to how scars form.

Scleroderma most frequently affects the skin, but it can also affect the gastrointestinal tract, lungs, kidneys, heart, blood vessels, muscles, and joints. In its most severe forms, scleroderma can be fatal.

Scleroderma affects about 250 adults per million in the United States. It typically appears between the ages of 30 and 50, but there is also a pediatric form. Women are four times more likely than men to have scleroderma. At the point when a safe reaction fools tissues into thinking they are harmed, it causes aggravation, and the body makes an excess of collagen, prompting scleroderma. An excess of collagen in your skin and different tissues causes patches of tight, hard skin. Numerous body systems are involved in scleroderma. The accompanying definitions can assist you with a better comprehension of what sickness means for every one of those frameworks.

Scleroderma is a very rare condition. Its commonness fluctuates with identity, orientation, and geographic region. In 2002, it was estimated that 158.3 people per million people in France had systemic sclerosis, mostly in cutaneous forms. Between 1989 and 1991, the disease had a prevalence of 242 cases per million adults in Detroit, with 19.3 new cases per million adults each year. Women are more likely than men to suffer from autoimmune diseases (ratio 4.6:1). Any age can experience systemic scleroderma; However, it only occurs in very affluent and young people. The disease affects most people between the ages of 30 and 50.

Confined scleroderma influences generally ladies with a frequency of 3 cases for every 100,000 people/year. Plaque structure (additionally called morphea) is more common in grown-ups while straight scleroderma influences for the most part youngsters

A connective tissue infection is one that influences tissues like skin, ligaments, and ligaments. Connective tissue upholds, secures, and gives design to different tissues and organs.
Immune system illnesses happen when the safe framework, which regularly shields the body from contamination and illness, goes

after its own tissues. A group of conditions known as rheumatic diseases are characterized by pain or inflammation in the muscles, joints, or fibrous tissue.

Scleroderma does not have a treatment. The treatment aims to stop the disease from getting worse and relieve symptoms. Important factors include early diagnosis and ongoing monitoring.

Scleroderma has no known cause. However, researchers believe that the immune system overreacts, causing blood vessel cells to become inflamed and injured. This triggers connective tissue cells, particularly a phone type called fibroblasts, to make a lot of collagen and different proteins. Fibroblasts live longer than ordinary, causing the development of collagen in the skin and different organs, prompting the signs and side effects of scleroderma. Scleroderma is brought about by three primary mechanisms: vascular irregularities, abundance fibrosis, and immune system peculiarity.

The involvement of the microcirculatory vascular system is caused by abnormal interactions between endothelial cells, fibroblasts, and lymphocytes (B and T). The endothelial cells produce a lot of endothelin 1, causing vasoconstriction and fibroblast enactment. In addition, activated endothelial cells and fibroblasts produce reactive oxygen species that accelerate vascular remodeling and eliminate small vessels. Myofibroblasts, which are capable of producing more collagen, are easily differentiated from activated fibroblasts.

The joining structure "sclero" signifies "hard" in Greek, and "dermis" signifies skin.

Types of scleroderma:
There are two primary types of scleroderma: localized and systemic [also called systemic sclerosis (SSc)].

In localized scleroderma, the sickness influences chiefly the skin and may affect the muscles and bones. Localized scleroderma, the disease's more common form, only affects a person's skin, usually in a few places. It frequently manifests itself on the skin as waxy streaks or patches, and it is not uncommon for the less severe form to disappear or cease to progress without treatment.

1. Systemic scleroderma:
In systemic scleroderma, There is involvement of the internal organs, including the heart, lungs, kidneys, digestive system, and others. Scleroderma can be severe or treatable in a variety of ways. Systemic scleroderma can sometimes become serious and life-threatening.
Scleroderma of the system can be divided into two main categories: diffuse and limited scleroderma.

However, most patients do not have all the symptoms described below.
Raynaud's phenomenon
After being exposed to cold or a change in temperature, Raynaud's phenomenon (RP)

is secondary to vasospasm in the proximal arteries. It is the most considered normal appearance of foundational sclerosis, happening in over 95% of patients. There are three phases to the typical RP crisis: syncopal paleness with sedation restricted to a couple of fingers, cyanosis paresthesia, and late erythematous, difficult stage.

Raynaud's phenomenon causes specific pieces of your body, generally the fingers, toes, ears, or tip of your nose to feel cold and go numb in chilly temperatures or when you feel worried. Your skin might turn blue after turning white. As the bloodstream gets back to business as usual, the impacted regions frequently become red. Not every person with Raynaud's has scleroderma. Scleroderma patients, on the other hand, may encounter issues as a result of restricted blood flow. The skin on the fingers can be damaged by Raynaud's, resulting in sores or pits.

RP is frequently complicated by trophic conditions, particularly digital ulcers. At least one episode of digital ulceration will occur in approximately half of patients with systemic scleroderma. Distal gangrene, which may necessitate an auto-amputation, can develop as a result of digital ischemia. Nailfold capillaroscopy reveals architectural disorganization, giant capillaries, hemorrhages, loss of capillaries, angiogenesis, and avascular areas in more than 95% of patients with SSc.

(a) Diffuse scleroderma;
This form has a wide range of effects on the body, as its name suggests. It can have an effect not only on the skin but also on a number of internal organs, making it difficult to breathe and digest food and can even lead to kidney failure. Diffuse scleroderma is a subtype of scleroderma where overabundance collagen creation causes skin thickening over a huge region of the body, typically the fingers, hands, arms,

front trunk, legs and face. There can be critical related organ harm, including to the gastrointestinal parcel, kidneys, lungs and heart.

(b) Limited scleroderma;
Limited scleroderma is the most well-known kind of scleroderma. Skin tightening and hardening usually only affects the fingers, but it can also affect the face, hands, or forearms. The limited scleroderma type is less likely to cause damage to internal organs. Patients with limited scleroderma typically live normal lives. Some suffer from digestive issues, particularly heartburn; severe musculoskeletal and Raynaud's pain; likewise, a small subset may develop potentially fatal pulmonary hypertension.

A subtype of limited scleroderma is also known as CREST syndrome. CREST is an acronym for its most prominent clinical features, each letter stands for a feature of the disease:

C - Calcinosis (abnormal calcium deposits in the skin)

R - Raynaud's phenomenon (exaggerated response to ambient temperatures making the skin of the fingers or toes cold, numb or tingling with color changes)

E - Esophageal dysmotility (difficulty swallowing)

S - Sclerodactyly (skin tightening on the fingers)

T - Telangiectasias (red spots on the skin)

There are no kidney issues in those with limited scleroderma. The skin thickening is confined to the fingers, hands, and lower arms, and furthermore some of the time the feet and legs. The esophagus is the primary site of digestive involvement. Pulmonary hypertension, which can develop in 20% to 30% of cases, is one of the later complications that can be potentially serious. In pulmonary hypertension, the arteries that connect the heart to the lungs narrow, putting a lot of pressure on the right side of the heart, and this can eventually result in right-sided heart failure. Early side effects of respiratory hypertension incorporate windedness, chest torment, and weariness

2. Localized scleroderma:
Scleroderma localized typically progresses through three distinct phases: edematous, indurated, and sclerotic, and then atrophic. Its result is unusual and unconstrained upgrades are conceivable. In the same patient, multiple clinical manifestations of localized scleroderma can coexist. Localized scleroderma is broken down into two main categories: morphea and scleroderma linear.

(a) Morphea scleroderma;
Morphea is the most well-known clinical structure. It presents as a solitary or different plaque. These plaques begin as erythematous before transforming into sclerosis, white, indurated, and surrounded by a distinctive erythematous halo known as

a "purple ring" to indicate their inflammatory activity. Although pruritus may be present, the pain is generally absent. Hypopigmentation develops later, and the lesions generally become atrophic. The trunk and proximal extremities are primarily affected by the lesions; Rarely is the face affected.

Plaque morphea can additionally arrange into other subtypes, as indicated by the shape or profundity of the sores. " Guttate" morphea or "white spot sickness" alludes to "drop-like" molded areas of skin contribution, though "subcutaneous" or profound morphea demonstrates a significant inclusion of more profound tissues with a relative saving of the overlying skin.

Although the subcutaneous type rarely penetrates muscle, this does not necessarily indicate the involvement of internal organs.

Generalized morphea is characterized as different morphea plaques, intersecting or not, influencing multiple physical locales. Bullous morphea is an uncommon sub-type portrayed by rankles or disintegrations happening on plaques of morphea.

Circumscribed Morphea
With circumscribed morphea (one more name for stained patches of skin), you might have a solitary oval fix or you might see a couple of patches of morphea. The patches fluctuate in size and commonly have a red line and a thickened light yellow place. These injuries can augment when dynamic and afterward level and become asymptomatic with treatment. Profound outlined morphea stretches out into the subcutaneous tissues.

(b) Linear scleroderma;
Linear scleroderma appears as thickened and indurated skin groups, which are most

frequently on the face or limits. It is the most normal type of scleroderma in kids.

On the scalp or face, linear scleroderma gives a perspective called "en upset de saber" (a French demeanor signifying "cut from a blade"). The sclerotic band is by and large situated on the brow yet can stretch out to the scalp (causing scarring alopecia), and to the nose as well as the upper lip.

The skin is hypo or hyperpigmented, atrophic, and sticks to the hidden bone. This type of scleroderma is hard to distinguish from Parry-Romberg syndrome because it frequently occurs in conjunction with ipsilateral hemiatrophy of the face.

Linear scleroderma of the appendages is classified as "monomelic" and frequently starts in youth. Sclero-atrophic groups show up slowly and afterward stretch out to the muscles and ligaments; This could result in a severe form of pansclerotic morphea with joint and bone deformities and limb stoppage or retardation of growth.

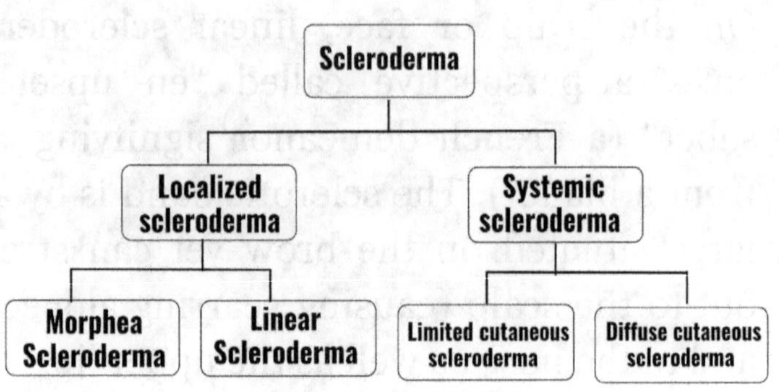

Types of Scleroderma

Causes and Risk Factors:

Scleroderma's exact cause is unknown. Albeit once in a long while, scleroderma can run in families. Most cases show no family background of the illness. Scleroderma does not spread.

Scleroderma's causes are not completely understood. Scleroderma's genesis may be influenced by genetic and environmental factors, according to some evidence. Silica and certain natural solvents are perceived as hazardous elements of an event of fundamental scleroderma. The immune system becomes activated, causing tissue damage and damage to blood vessels, which in turn causes scar tissue and the accumulation of excessive collagen.

At the very least, genetic factors play a small role. Scleroderma was found in 13 times more first-degree relatives of scleroderma patients than in the general population, according to three US cohort studies. OX40L quality polymorphism connects with fundamental scleroderma. IRF5 quality was found to relate with fundamental scleroderma as well likewise with the event of interstitial lung infection during scleroderma.

Anybody can get scleroderma; in any case, a few gatherings have a higher risk of fostering the sickness. Your risk may be affected by the following factors.

Gender: It affects women significantly more than men. Upwards of 80% of those determined to have scleroderma are ladies.

Age: The disease is more prevalent in adults than in children and typically manifests between the ages of 30 and 50.

Race: All races and ethnic groups can get scleroderma, but African Americans are more likely to get it. For instance:

African Americans are more likely than European Americans to be affected by the disease.

African Americans with scleroderma foster the illness prior when contrasted and different gatherings. When compared to other groups, African Americans are more likely to have lung disease and skin involvement.

Ecological openness: Scleroderma can be made more likely in some people by certain factors in the environment. Scleroderma appears to be more common in men exposed to silica. Being around sure solvents and consuming specific medications can likewise build your true capacity for fostering the illness.

Genes: Hereditary qualities assume a part in the illness, however, it isn't given from guardians to youngsters, and it's uncommon for close relatives of those with scleroderma to get it. However, family members frequently suffer from other autoimmune conditions like lupus, rheumatoid arthritis, or thyroid disease. Scleroderma may be more likely for you if you have a particular gene makeup. There is evidence that SS affects parents, siblings, and children more frequently. The most noteworthy commonness of SS in the US is among a Local American clan known as the Oklahoma Choctaw Indians, where they experience 469 cases for every 100,000 individuals. This older statistic may provide additional support for the possibility that genetics play a significant role in SS.

Hormones: Ladies foster most kinds of scleroderma more frequently than men. The disease may be influenced by hormonal differences between men and women, according to researchers.

Exposure to certain agents may trigger SS, including:

Infections, medications, drugs, synthetics, Invulnerable framework issues, Since scleroderma is an immune system condition, it might happen because your insusceptible framework obliterates your connective tissues. The following connective tissue disorders are thought to be present in 15 to 25% of people with SS: polymyositis, dermatomyositis, rheumatoid joint inflammation, Sjögren's illness — Sjögren's disorder is caused by dry eyes and mouth. The immune system's destruction of the body's moisture-producing glands results in a lack of tears and saliva, which causes this dryness. Henrik Sjögren, a Swedish eye doctor who first described this condition, is credited with giving it its name. It affects approximately 20% of scleroderma patients.

Esophageal brokenness, which alludes to the debilitated capability of the throat (the cylinder associating the throat and the stomach) that happens when smooth muscles in the throat lose ordinary development. Sclerodactyly is thick, tight skin on the fingers caused by deposits of too much collagen in the layers of the skin.

Telangiectasia is a condition in which small blood vessels swell, resulting in red spots on the hands and face.

Diffuse cutaneous scleroderma comes on abruptly, typically with skin thickening on the fingers or toes. After that, the skin thickens all over the body, above the elbows and/or knees. This kind can hurt your internal organs: anywhere in the digestive tract. the heart, kidneys, and lungs.

Chapter 2

Clinical manifestations:
Lesions of the skin are bilateral and symmetrical, beginning distally on the fingers and occasionally on the toes. Two

distinct clinical characteristics should be distinguished.

Diffuse SSc, which affects 30 to 40 percent of patients and causes cutaneous sclerosis to rise above the elbows and knees.

During limited SSc, the cutaneous involvement is restricted to the face, hands, fingers, and forearms. Sclerotic lesions may appear several months before swelled fingers and hands. Additionally, the skin on the fingers appears tense, giving the impression of being "sausage-like." The skin of the fingers becomes dry, thick, and harsh to the touch: This condition, known as sclerodactyly, makes it difficult to form a fist with the hand.

The nails shrink, curl, and occasionally vanish. The skin becomes waxy and the folds fade, giving the face an unimpressive appearance. The lips and nose are thin. Skin xerosis causes the skin around the lips to develop smaller, finer wrinkles. Consumption of solid foods, dental care, and other activities may be restricted as a result

of the restricted oral opening. The distance between the incisors is used to measure one's capacity to open the mouth. During SSc, telangiectasias are common and typically occur in the face and mucous membranes.
Other cutaneous signs such as calcinosis, pigmentation disorders, and telangiectasia may be present.

The Modified Rodnan Skin Score measures the importance and extent of cutaneous sclerosis in 17 body regions (0: normal thickness of the skin; 1: very little thickening; 2: moderate thickening; 3: major thickening). In diffuse structures, this score has a prognostic worth, and for the most part arrives at its greatest in the initial three years after Raynaud's peculiarity and afterward will in general improve immediately.

Pulmonary impairment;

The pulmonary lesions include interstitial lung disease (ILD) and pulmonary arterial hypertension (PAH). These two complications are the leading causes of death during SSc.

Pulmonary arterial hypertension;
Systemic scleroderma patients can have up to 13% of them develop pulmonary arterial hypertension (PAH). Patients with limited cutaneous systemic sclerosis are more likely to experience it. PAH is, by definition, pulmonary arterial pressure measured by right catheterization at rest that is greater than or equal to 25 mmHg. PAH is thought when aspiratory blood vessel systolic strain surpasses 40 mm Hg very still in echocardiography. Patients can go a long time without showing any symptoms, especially if they don't do a lot of physical activity. Signs of seriousness include syncope, hemoptysis, and dysphonia (Ortner's syndrome). A loud second heart sound, signs of right heart failure, and a

systolic or diastolic murmur of tricuspid insufficiency may be detected during an examination.

Interstitial lung disease (ILD);
Interstitial lung Disease (ILD) is normal in patients with SSc since up to 90% of patients show proof of interstitial changes on high-goal registered tomography (HRCT). With the disease's diffuse forms, it occurs more frequently. Crackles in the bases can be seen through pulmonary auscultation in patients with or without dyspnea and dry cough. ILD evaluation is by aspiratory capability tests (PFTs) and HRCT. Ground-glass images are the most common, followed by septal or intralobular images, linear or reticular images, and a honeycomb appearance with traction bronchiectasis. SSc-ILD shows up in the early long stretches of the sickness, and its most stamped movement happens in the principal years after conclusion. ILD movement is generally sluggish; However,

respiratory failure can develop in about 12% of scleroderma patients. Poorer survival is correlated with an ILD affecting more than 20% of the lung parenchyma.

Gastrointestinal manifestations;
The entire digestive tract is involved in SSc's gastrointestinal involvement. In between 75 and 90% of patients, gastroesophageal reflux disease (GERD) occurs. Erosive esophagitis, peptic stenosis, and endo-brachy-esophagus should all be ruled out if a patient complains of dysphagia. Additionally, motor impairment can affect the stomach, resulting in gastroparesis and, less frequently, watermelon stomach, which is a condition associated with gastric antral vascular ectasia. The motor impairment causes bacterial overgrowth in the small intestine, as well as nutritional deficiencies (vitamin B12 and folate), malabsorption (steatorrhea), and pseudo-obstruction. Fecal incontinence and rectal prolapse may result from anorectal involvement.

Cardiac manifestations;

They are normal in SSc. Be that as it may, just 15% of patients are suggestive and afterward have an unfortunate forecast (assessed 2-year mortality: 60%). Myocardial disease, defects in the conduction system, arrhythmias, and pericardial disease are all examples of cardiac involvement.

Most of the time, only the microcirculation of the heart is affected. On account of respiratory infection, the right cardiovascular breakdown is conceivable. Pericardial contribution is very normal during SSc, generally without clinical results. Conduction issues are very interesting. Holter-electrocardiogram can detect disorders of the heart's rhythm.

Renal involvement;

Patients with SSc frequently have involvement in the Kidney. The most serious sign is scleroderma renal crisis (SRC) which is an interesting but significant inconvenience. It distinctively shows the event of unexpected beginning hypertension and oligo/anuric intense renal disappointment. Malignant hypertension is characterized by clinical symptoms. SRC is more normal in patients with diffuse SSc and hostility to RNA-polymerase III antibodies. SRC was the most common fatal complication of systemic scleroderma prior to the use of angiotensin-converting enzyme (ACE) inhibitors.

Musculoskeletal Manifestations;
Scleroderma might influence joints (joint inflammation, arthralgia), ligaments (rubs, tenosynovitis), and muscles (myalgia, shortcoming, all the more seldom myositis). A poor outcome is indicated by friction tendon rubs on the hands, knees, and ankles. Major functional disorders can result from digital retractions in flexion caused by skin sclerosis and calcinosis.
Alternative Names

Progressive systemic sclerosis; Systemic sclerosis; Limited scleroderma; CREST syndrome; Localized scleroderma; Morphea - linear; Raynaud's phenomenon - scleroderma

Scleroderma has many signs and symptoms such as:
Skin that is hard, thickening, or tight is what gives scleroderma its name. A few individuals develop hard, thick skin patches. Others have broad patches on their body.
The thick, hard skin can appear to be stuck in place. The patches may not feel too hard if you have morphea (more-fee-uh), the most common type of scleroderma. The hardened skin may soften over time.

☐ Hair loss and less sweating.
You will frequently notice hair loss and shiny, discolored skin where you have hardened skin. The skin that has hardened often also loses the ability to sweat.

☐ Dry skin and itch.

Scleroderma causes extremely dry skin to itch and becomes extremely dry. The skin may break down and develop sores as a result of extreme dryness.

☐ Skin color changes.

The patches of hardened skin can be lighter or darker than your natural skin color. Some people develop violet-colored skin, which means that the scleroderma is active and expanding.

☐ Salt-and-pepper look to the skin.

On the upper back, chest, or scalp (along the hairline), this usually appears. Sometimes, the skin may feel hard or tight. If you have a salt-and-pepper look on your skin, you ought to see a specialist. This may indicate that you have internal organ-affecting scleroderma. Your prognosis—what is likely to happen is better the sooner you are diagnosed and treated.

☐ Stiff joints and difficulty moving them.
At the point when the hard, thickening, or tight skin structures over a joint (i.e., the jaw, wrist, or finger), the snugness can make it challenging to move that joint. Active recuperation can assist you with keeping the full scope of movement. Without it, you might lose the capacity to completely fix or curve a finger, elbow, wrist, or other piece of your body.

☐ Muscle shortening and weakness.
The solidifying and tightening at times reaches out to the muscle. The muscle may become short and weak as a result. The muscle may not be able to be stretched. It is essential to inform your doctor if you experience muscle weakness so that the underlying cause can be identified and treated.

☐ Loss of tissue beneath the skin.
Parry-Romberg syndrome (PRS) is the name given to this kind of scleroderma,

which can result in the breakdown of bone, cartilage, and muscle. Most of the time, PRS affects one side of the face. It can also affect the trunk, arm, or leg. PRS rarely occurs. The loss of tissue beneath the skin can also occur in other forms of scleroderma.

☐ Bone may not grow as it should.
Some kinds of scleroderma, like linear scleroderma or en coup de sabre, can make it hard for a child to grow bones. A leg may not create as it ought to. On the off chance that scleroderma influences the head, the face might become disfigured. These malformations are uncommon.

☐ Sores and pitted scars on the fingers.
Skin sores are common in people who have a type of scleroderma that also affects the internal organs. The skin that is tightly stretched is more likely to develop these sores. On the fingers, sores are especially common. On their fingertips and the sides

of their fingers, some people develop pitted scars the size of pinheads.

☐ Calcium deposits beneath the skin
Calcinosis (pronounced KAL-sin-OH-sis) is a condition that affects the connective tissue beneath the skin. Under your skin, you might feel one or more painful, hard lumps. You'll see a white or yellow chalky substance if a calcium deposit breaks through the skin. This can be very painful. It's possible for an infection and painful open sores to form. Extreme sensitivity to cold, stress, or both is frequently an early sign that the internal organs are affected by scleroderma.

How scleroderma is diagnosed:
Experts who most generally break down scleroderma are dermatologists and rheumatologists. Rheumatologists center around illnesses that influence the joints, muscles, and bones, while dermatologists are specialists in diagnosing skin-related conditions.

Scleroderma is typically diagnosed by asking you about your symptoms, health, and medical history. Your skin will also be examined by the doctor for signs of thickening and hardening.

On the off chance that you have hard, thickened skin, a dermatologist could play out a skin biopsy to help with diagnosing you. This quick and easy test can be performed by your dermatologist during an office visit. Your dermatologist will wipe out a bit of affected skin so it might be reviewed under an amplifying instrument.

Scleroderma diagnosis is not always straightforward. Since it can influence different pieces of the body, for example, the joints, scleroderma might be at first confused with rheumatoid joint pain or lupus.

Your doctor will conduct a comprehensive physical examination after discussing your personal and family medical history. As part of this process, he or she will be looking for any of the aforementioned symptoms, particularly thickening or hardening of the skin around the fingers and toes or skin discoloration. In the event that scleroderma is thought of, tests will be requested to affirm the determination, as well as to decide the seriousness of the illness. Some of these tests might be:

Blood tests:
Raised levels of resistant components, known as antinuclear antibodies, are seen in 95% of patients with scleroderma. Even though these antibodies are additionally found in other immune system illnesses like lupus, testing for them in individuals who could have scleroderma makes it more straightforward to make a decent finding.

Pulmonary function tests:
The purpose of these tests is to assess how well the lungs are working. Checking to see if scleroderma has spread to the lungs, where it can cause scar tissue to form, is

critical if scleroderma is suspected or confirmed. To check for damage to the lungs, an X-ray or a computed tomography (CT) scan may be used.

Electrocardiogram:
Heart tissue scarring caused by scleroderma can lead to congestive heart failure and inadequate electrical movement of the heart. This test is finished to check whether the heart has been impacted by the infection. An ultrasonogram of the heart called an echocardiogram: This should be done once every six to 12 months to check for complications like pulmonary hypertension and/or congestive heart failure.

Gastrointestinal tests:
Both the throat muscles and the digestive tract walls can be impacted by scleroderma. This can affect how supplements are retained in the body and how food moves through the digestive tract, as well as lead to problems with gulping and acid reflux. By

inserting a small tube with a camera on the end, manometry, a test that measures the strength of the esophageal muscles, can also be used to view the esophagus and intestines.

Kidney function:
Scleroderma can affect the kidneys, allowing protein to leak into the urine and raising blood pressure. In its most serious design (called scleroderma renal crisis), a quick extension in heartbeat could occur, achieving kidney dissatisfaction. Blood tests can be used to assess kidney capacity.

Chapter 3

Treatment Approaches:
As of now, there is no remedy for scleroderma. All things being equal, treatment is aimed at controlling and dealing with the side effects. To effectively treat and manage scleroderma, a variety of treatments are frequently required due to the disease's numerous symptoms.

Skin treatments: For localized scleroderma, skin meds frequently are valuable. Creams are utilized to keep the skin from drying out, as well as to treat solidified skin. Nitrates like nitroglycerin are prescribed to increase blood flow and speed up the healing process for finger abrasions. Nitrates work by loosening up the smooth muscles, making the conduits expand (broaden). Generally, smooth muscles are those that support some internal organs and blood vessels. Consult your doctor before taking nitrates because they can cause side effects like dizziness, nausea, rapid heartbeat, and blurred vision.

Digestive remedies:
Different prescriptions might be recommended to assist patients with indigestion and other stomach-related Issues. These incorporate over-the-counter and recommended acid neutralizers, proton siphon inhibitors, and H2 receptor blockers. Proton pump inhibitors prevent stomach acid from being secreted by inhibiting the proton or acid pump. H2 receptor blockers work by blocking histamine, a chemical in

the body that makes the stomach produce more acid.

Treatment of lung disease:
In a recent NIH study, the drug cyclophosphamide, a type of chemotherapy, was found to be beneficial for patients with scleroderma who also had rapidly worsening pulmonary fibrosis or scarring of the lung tissue. In scleroderma patients with interstitial lung disease, this study demonstrated that oral cyclophosphamide improved lung function and quality of life.
The most effective treatment for pulmonary hypertension is continuous intravenous infusion of epoprostenol, a prostaglandin, via a pump. The subcutaneous mixture of treprostinil, a connected prostaglandin, is a satisfactory other option. Prostaglandins are hormone-like substances found in the body. They help relax smooth muscle and, as a result, widen blood vessels. Oral bosentan, sildenafil, and inhaled iloprost are other

treatments for pulmonary hypertension that are currently approved by the FDA.

Pulmonary hypertension and severe (drug-refractory) interstitial lung disease can both benefit from a lung transplant.

Joint difficulties: For patients with scleroderma who experience joint issues, mitigating medications might be recommended. These medications work by diminishing aggravation and thus the pain and expanding. Occasionally, physical therapy to stop joints from contracting can be helpful.

Raynaud's phenomenon: Vasodilators like calcium channel blockers, nitroglycerin patches, ointments, alpha-blockers like sildenafil, and so on are all effective treatments. Aspirin and other antiplatelet medications are frequently added. Oral medications like sildenafil or the preventative use of bosentan can be helpful for ischemic digital ulcers. For fingers with serious ulceration or looming gangrene, hospitalization for a preliminary intravenous epoprostenol or alprostadil is fitting. Contaminated ulcers need neighborhood wound care and a drawn-out course of fitting anti-infection agents.

Sjögren's syndrome: The symptoms can be alleviated, but there is no cure. Dry eyes can be treated with counterfeit tears and cyclosporine eye drops. A dry mouth can be eased by tasting fluids or biting gum. In additional extreme instances of dry mouth, sedates that animate the development of spit might be endorsed.

Kidney problems: Scleroderma-related kidney problems can be managed and treated with medication, particularly angiotensin-converting enzyme (ACE) inhibitors, and dialysis, depending on the severity of the condition.

Other things that help may include:

Keeping your muscles strong through exercise and physical therapy, eating more fiber and fluids, getting treatment for your skin, such as light and laser therapy, managing your stress, and getting an organ transplant if your organs are badly damaged.

Your skin is the biggest organ of your body, composed of a few distinct parts, including water, protein, lipids, and various minerals and synthetic substances. Its occupation is urgent: to shield you from infections and other threats posed by the environment. The skin likewise contains nerves that sense cold, heat, torment, strain, and contact.
All through your life, your skin will change continually, no matter what. In point of fact, your skin will regenerate itself about once per month. To keep this organ's health and vitality intact, proper skin care is essential.

Layers of the Skin There are layers to the skin. It comprises a flimsy external layer (epidermis), a thicker center layer (dermis), and the internal layer (subcutaneous tissue or hypodermis).

Epidermis: The External Layer of Skin
The external layer of skin, the epidermis, is a clear layer made of cells that capability to shield us from the climate. The most superficial layer is made up of constantly shed dead skin cells. Basal cells that are responsible for skin renewal are found in the deepest part. Keratin, a protein made inside the cells of the epidermis, safeguards the skin from harmful substances, like compound items and microorganisms. Additionally, melanin-producing cells are located in the epidermis. The epidermis is liable for the look and strength of the skin and it holds a lot of water. The skin contains more water the younger the body. With age, the skin's ability to retain water decreases, making it more susceptible to dehydration. Keratin is the skin's strongest protein.

Additionally, it strengthens the hair and nails.

Dermis: The Dermis' Middle Layer consists of two types of fibers that become scarcer with age: collagen, which gives skin its strength, and elastin, which gives skin its elasticity. Blood and lymph vessels, hair follicles, sweat glands, and oil-producing sebaceous glands are all found in the dermis. Nerves in the dermis sense contact and agony. The skin's most abundant protein is collagen. 75% of your skin is covered in it. This is likewise your "wellspring of youth," answerable for warding off kinks and almost negligible differences. Your body's capacity to produce collagen deteriorates over time due to aging and environmental factors. Elastin, which is found in the same place as collagen, gives your organs and skin their structure. Similarly, as with collagen, elastin is impacted by time and the components.

Reduced levels of this protein make your skin flaw and droop.

Hypodermis: The Fatty Layer The hypodermis, or subcutaneous tissue, is primarily composed of fat. It contains blood vessels that expand and contract to help maintain a constant body temperature and is located between the dermis and muscles or bones. Your vital internal organs are also protected by the hypodermis. Your skin will sag as the tissue in this layer shrinks.

Sweat glands and sebaceous glands The sebaceous glands produce sebum, an oily substance that prevents skin from becoming dry. Sebum decreases water misfortune from the skin surface, safeguards the skin from contamination by microbes and parasites, and adds to the stench. These organs are connected to hair follicles.
The sweat glands in your body produce sweat, which evaporates to keep you cool when you're hot or under stress. There are

sweat glands all over the body, but your palms, soles, forehead, and underarms have the most. When the fluid comes into contact with bacteria that are typically found on your skin, the specialized sweat glands known as the apocrine glands produce an odor.

Chronic scleroderma can affect a person's mental and physical well-being at the same time. The best way to feel better with scleroderma is to tailor the treatment to the patient's specific needs, taking into account their symptoms, type of scleroderma, age, and overall health. The above accentuation on skin types and functions will assist you with understanding the sort of side effects you are encountering on your body.

Because scleroderma can affect a lot of important aspects of life, it's important to have a trusted team to help you deal with challenges. Patients may require assistance from family and friends at various points in time or from specialists like a physical therapist or personal assistant.

Since scleroderma can change your appearance and make it challenging to do ordinary assignments, it could cause pressure and stress more than expected. As stress can influence the seriousness of the infection, learning strategies for adapting to this condition is significant. Specialists frequently utilize a reference to an instructor or a scleroderma support group.

The Long-Term Prognosis for Scleroderma;
Numerous scleroderma patients, even those with more intrusive foundational scleroderma, can hope to have an ordinary future. In any case, to stay as sound as could be expected, you should open up to the specialist about how you feel. Your doctor should keep a close eye on your health and address any issues as soon as they arise.

There are a number of specific issues that are important to consider:

There may be a time when some patients' conditions improve. Their skin may get better and their mobility may get better during this time. This might change quickly or even go into long-term remission.

Monitoring: Screenings for internal organ complications should be performed regularly in patients with systemic scleroderma.

Pregnancy: Patients can get pregnant; Nonetheless, there is probably a greater chance of miscarriage. During pregnancy, a portion of the side effects (like Raynaud peculiarity) could improve, however, others (like indigestion) could deteriorate.

Living with scleroderma (Management);
A person with scleroderma can better manage the disease by taking several different actions, in addition to taking their prescribed medications on time and in the correct dosage. These include:

Exercise
Your overall physical and spiritual well-being will benefit from regular exercise, as will the flexibility and circulation of your joints. For exercises that are right for you, talk to your doctor or physical therapist.

Here are some Physiotherapy workouts for scleroderma
Many individuals track down physiotherapy as amazingly valuable in their battle against the side effects of scleroderma. The following are a few simple activities for the region of the body that many view as the most valuable to assist with overseeing pain and further developing portability.

1. Face:
When performed in front of a mirror, most people find these exercises easier. If you do these while your skin is warm, like after a hot shower or bath, you will stretch better. Alternatively, before stretching, you could

use a warm flannel to massage the face. To be effective, stretches should be performed three times per day and held for at least ten seconds. A double benefit is that many people find that strengthening facial muscles also prevents aging. Lower the eyebrows after raising them. Crush your eyes shut firmly. Wink firmly with one or the other eye. Grimace your forehead to wrinkle the extension of your nose, and raise your upper lip to expand the stretch. Flare up your nose. Close your lips hard. Open your mouth as wide as you can while covering your teeth with your lips. Bristle some fur and open your mouth to the furthest extent that you would be able. To create an underbite, move the jaw forward. While not displaying your teeth, grin as widely as you can.

2. Back:
Mid back twists - To feel a stretch in the middle of the back, twist to one side while sitting in a chair.

Low back rolling: Roll your knees gently from side to side while lying on your back on the bed with your knees bent together. Stretch with your hands behind your back: Holding onto a stick, place your hands behind your back and pull the stick up with your upper hand to stretch your lower arm. With your palm facing outward, Rehash for the opposite side. This stretch can be performed sitting down with a towel in place of the stick if it is simpler.

3. Neck:

Neck side flexions - Make sure not to look backward during this stretch, and tilt the head so that the ear is closer to the shoulder. You ought to feel a firm yet agreeable stretch at the contrary side of the neck, running down towards the shoulder.

Neck rotation: While seated, turn the head to the side and look over the shoulder without looking up or down. You ought to feel a firm however agreeable stretch on the contrary side of the neck to which you are looking.

4. Wrists:

Wrist extension stretch -Place your palms together and then lower them down your chest, keeping the palms' bases as close together as possible, until you feel a firm but comfortable stretch at your wrists' insides.
Wrist flexion stretch - Place the backs of your hands together and afterward lower them down the chest, keeping the foundation of the backs of the hands as near one another as conceivable until you feel a firm yet agreeable stretch beyond the wrists.

5. Shoulders:

Shoulder abduction stretch - Hold a stick, such as a walking stick, umbrella, golf club, or rolling pin, with the palms facing upward while standing. To feel the stretch, raise one arm to your side until you feel it. Rehash for the opposite side. This stretch can be done while sitting if that makes it easier.

Joint protection;
When your joints hurt, don't lift heavy objects or do things that could put a strain on them and put you at risk of getting hurt again. An actual specialist can assist you with learning better approaches to perform day to day exercises without overburdening your joints.

Skin protection;
Playing it safe and taking care of your skin can be useful for side effects of Raynaud's phenomenon, yet additionally in dealing with the dry, thick fixes of skin that outcome from localized scleroderma.

This can be accomplished in a variety of ways, including:
Dressing appropriately during the colder months. Boots, a hat, gloves, and a scarf will help keep your extremities' blood vessels open and your circulation flowing while also keeping your body warm and protected from

the cold. Put on several thin layers. Rather than wearing just one thick layer, these will keep you warmer. To keep the blood flowing to your feet, wear boots or shoes with a loose fit. Put a humidifier in your home to assist with keeping the air wet.

Make use of creams and soaps that are made specifically for dry skin.

Diet;

Besides eating quality food sources to get legitimate measures of nutrients and supplements, it is essential to eat food sources that don't irritate existing stomach issues. Examples of this include:

1. Staying away from food sources that cause indigestion.

2. Drinking water or one more fluid to mellow food further.

3. consuming foods high in fiber to prevent constipation.

Eating more, more modest dinners rather than three enormous feasts. This makes it easier for the body to break down the food. Wait at least four hours before lying down if you have eaten a large meal. By placing blocks or bricks underneath the head of your bed, you can raise it by approximately six inches. This will keep the stomach corrosive from entering the throat while you are resting.

	Foods to be Consumed	Foods to be avoided
Fruits	Banana, Dates, watermelon, musk melon, figs, pomegranate, custard apple, peach, plum, guava, sapodilla, apple.	Orange, lime, berries, sour grapes, lemons, kiwi, mangoes.
Vegetable	Lettuce, broccoli, carrots, sweet potatoes, turnip, chicory greens, kale, spinach, beans, cabbage, Brussels, beet,	Tomatoes, brinjal, onion, garlic, ginger.

	cucumber, bell pepper, bottle gourd, bitter gourd, pumpkin.	
Grains	Brown rice, white rice, wheat, quinoa, millets.	Rye
Legumes	Chickpea, yellow lentils, green lentils.	Kidney beans, black grams, bengal grams.
Spices	Basil, oregano, rosemary, cinnamon, paprika, turmeric, cayenne, coriander, cumin, fenu-greek, cardamom, mustard, curry powder.	Black cardamom, carom seeds, clove, nutmeg, pimento.
Oils	Olive oil, almond oil, canola oil, soybean oil, rice bran oil.	Coconut oil
Nuts	Walnut, chia seeds, raisins, almond, pumpkin seeds, flax seeds, sunflower seeds.	Cashew, groundnuts, pistachio.

Diary products	Cow ghee	Milk butter, buttermilk, yogurt cord.
Beverage	Herbal tea, green tea, detox tea, coconut water, sugarcane juices, homemade soup, homemade juices.	Tea, coffee, alcohol, carbonated drinks, squashes canned soup.

Dental care: Proper dental care is essential for scleroderma patients who also have Sjögren's syndrome. Cavities and tooth decay are more likely to occur in people with Sjögren's syndrome.

Stress management: It is essential to acquire skills in stress management or reduction because the effects of stress can contribute to a decrease in blood flow and influence numerous other aspects of your health and emotions.

The following steps can be taken to accomplish this:

Getting enough rest and sleep. Whenever possible, avoid stressful situations. Eating a nutritious diet. Learning strategies to control nerves and fears. Exercising.

Despite the fact that scleroderma has no known cure, the condition is frequently manageable and progresses slowly, and those who suffer from it may live productive and healthy lives. In the same way as others different circumstances, schooling about scleroderma and nearby care groups can be the best apparatuses for dealing with the illness and decreasing the risk of additional entanglements.